FRAGILE X SYNDROME HANDBOOK

Beginners Comprehensive Guide To Dealing With Fragile X Syndrome

VINCENT JERRY

Table of Contents

Introductory

Fragile X syndrome (FXS) is a genetic disorder that results in a variety of intellectual and developmental impairments. It is one of the most prevalent inherited causes of intellectual impairment and autism spectrum disorder. Here are a few important details about Fragile X syndrome:

• FXS is caused by a mutation in the FMR1 gene, which is located on the X chromosome. The mutation occurs on one of the two X chromosomes that are typically present in humans. The mutation causes a deficiency in FMRP

(Fragile X Mental Retardation Protein), a protein that is essential for brain development and function.

• Intellectual and Developmental Disabilities Fragile X syndrome is frequently accompanied by a spectrum of intellectual and developmental disabilities. These can range in severity, but frequently include learning difficulties, cognitive impairment, and speech and language delays.

• Behavioral and Emotional Difficulties FXS is also associated with behavioral and emotional difficulties. Individuals with Fragile X syndrome may exhibit social anxiety, repetitive behaviors, hyperactivity, impulsivity, and sensory processing difficulties. Some people may also suffer from mood disorders, such as melancholy and anxiety.

• Although there are no distinct physical characteristics associated with FXS, some individuals may have subtle facial characteristics or connective tissue problems. In general, these physical characteristics are less pronounced than those seen in other genetic syndromes.

• Autism Spectrum Disorder (ASD): Many FXS patients also meet the diagnostic criteria for autism spectrum disorder (ASD). This means they may exhibit impaired social interactions, communication difficulties, and repetitive behaviors comparable to those observed in autism.

• The severity of FXS can differ significantly between affected individuals. Others may have intellectual and developmental disabilities of a more severe nature.

• The diagnosis of Fragile X syndrome is typically confirmed by genetic testing, which searches for mutations in the FMR1 gene. Also available is prenatal testing for families with a history of the disorder.

• Treatment and Support: Although there is no cure for FXS, early intervention and a multidisciplinary approach to treatment can assist affected individuals in reaching their maximum potential.

Individuals with FXS frequently receive speech therapy, occupational therapy, and behavioral interventions to address their unique requirements. To manage symptoms such as anxiety and hyperactivity, medications may also be prescribed.

- Families of individuals with Fragile X syndrome may benefit from gaining access to support services and resources, such as special education programs, support groups, and organizations devoted to FXS research and advocacy.

It is essential to note that FXS affects individuals differently, and each individual with the syndrome may experience unique challenges and strengths. Early diagnosis and appropriate interventions can make a substantial difference in the lives of individuals and families affected by Fragile X syndrome.

CHAPTER ONE
Fragile-X Syndrome Genetics

Fragile X syndrome (FXS) is caused by a mutation in a specific gene termed the FMR1 (Fragile X Mental Retardation 1) gene. Here is an overview of FXS's genetics:

• Location of the Gene: The FMR1 gene is found on the X chromosome. As a consequence, FXS is considered a genetic disorder linked to X. Individuals typically have either XX (female) or XY (male) chromosomes. The mutation is frequently detected on one of the X chromosomes in FXS.

• Repeat Expansion Mutation: The mutation that causes FXS is characterized by a sequence of three DNA nucleotides, CGG, that is repeated within the FMR1 gene. This CGG repeat region typically contains fewer than 45 repetitions in unaffected individuals. However, in individuals with FXS, this CGG repeat region is excessively expanded and can contain hundreds or even thousands of repeats.

• Methylation and FMRP: The number of CGG repeats in the FMR1 gene dictates the function of the gene. In individuals with a normal number of repeats, the FMR1 gene is active and produces a protein called FMRP (Fragile X Mental Retardation Protein), which is essential for the development and function of the brain.

When there is a substantial expansion of CGG repeats (typically more than 200 repeats) in individuals with FXS, the FMR1 gene becomes methylated. Methylation effectively "silences" the gene, resulting in a FMRP deficiency.

• Absence of FMRP: The absence or deficiency of FMRP resulting from a mutation in the FMR1 gene is the underlying cause of the cognitive and developmental impairments observed in FXS. FMRP is indispensable for synaptic plasticity, the mechanism by which neurons communicate and adapt to new information. Its absence disrupts the normal development of neural pathways and causes the cognitive and behavioral symptoms of FXS.

• Carrier Status: Individuals who possess a premutation in the FMR1 gene (between 45 and 200 CGG repeats) may not exhibit FXS symptoms, but they can transmit the expanded CGG repeat to their offspring.

This can lead to their offspring inheriting the complete mutation and FXS. In addition, premutation carriers may be at risk for developing adult-onset conditions known as Fragile X-associated Tremor/Ataxia Syndrome (FXTAS) or Fragile X-associated Primary Ovarian Insufficiency (FXPOI).

FXS is caused by an expansion of CGG repeats in the FMR1 gene on the X chromosome, leading to a deficiency of the FMRP protein. This deficiency disrupts normal brain development and function, resulting in intellectual and developmental disabilities as well as behavioral symptoms that are characteristic of Fragile X syndrome.

The genetic inheritance pattern of FXS is complex, with carrier parents potentially passing on the mutation to their offspring. Genetic testing is used to diagnose FXS and determine the carrier or affected status of an individual.

Fragile X syndrome (FXS) can manifest with a broad variety of signs and symptoms whose severity varies between affected individuals. Although not all individuals with FXS will exhibit every sign or symptom, the following are frequent manifestations of the syndrome:

1. Disabilities of Intellect and Development:

• Cognitive impairment, including intellectual disability in differing degrees.

• Speech and language development delays.

• Difficulties with abstract reasoning and solving problems.

2. Behavioral and Emotional Challenges:

• Social apprehension and difficulty interacting with others.

• Reticence and shyness in social situations.

• Repetitive behaviors, such as fluttering the hands or speaking repeatedly.

• Impulsivity and hyperactivity.

- Sensory sensitivities or sensory processing issues.

- Difficulty with routine alterations and transitions.

3. Communication Problems:

- Limited vocabulary and difficulty expressing thoughts and demands.

- Echolalia (words or phrases repeated without comprehension).

- Difficulties in comprehending and utilizing nonverbal communication signals.

4. Autism Spectrum Characteristics:

• Some FXS patients meet the diagnostic criteria for autism spectrum disorder (ASD), which is characterized by impaired social interactions, communication difficulties, and repetitive behaviors.

5. Physical and Health-Related Considerations:

• Mild to moderate physical characteristics, including a long visage, large ears, and a prominent jaw or forehead (though these characteristics are not as pronounced as they are in other genetic syndromes).

• Connective tissue disorders, such as hypermobility of the joints or flat feet.

• Epilepsy (seizures) occur in a minority of FXS patients.

• Gastrointestinal problems like reflux or irritable bowel syndrome may be present.

6. Problems with Focus and Hyperactivity:

• Symptoms resembling Attention-deficit hyperactivity disorder

(ADHD), including inattention, hyperactivity, and impulsivity.

7. Behavior and Emotional Disorders:

• Emotional lability, alterations in mood, and irritability.

• Nervousness and anxieties.

• Aggressive or self-destructive behaviors (although these are more prevalent in males with FXS).

8. Sensory Hypersensitivity:

• Sensitivity to sensory stimuli, such as sounds, lights, textures, and flavors, is heightened.

9. Sleep Disorders:

• Sleep disturbances, such as trouble falling asleep or remaining unconscious.

It is essential to note that the severity and combination of symptoms can vary greatly between FXS sufferers. Some people may have milder forms of the disorder and function at a higher level, whereas others may have more severe difficulties in multiple areas.

Early diagnosis and intervention, such as speech therapy, occupational therapy, behavioral therapy, and educational support, can substantially improve the quality of life and maximize the potential of individuals with Fragile X Syndrome (FXS). There are also supportive services and resources available to help individuals with FXS and their families manage the condition.

CHAPTER TWO
Evaluation And Screening

Fragile X syndrome (FXS) is typically diagnosed through a combination of clinical evaluation, genetic testing, and family history analysis. Here is a summary of the FXS diagnosis and screening process:

1. Clinical Evaluation:

• A pediatrician or clinical geneticist may initially suspect FXS based on a child's developmental and behavioral symptoms. These may include delays in speech and language, intellectual disabilities, social difficulties, and repetitive behaviors.

2. Family History Assessment:

• Collecting a thorough family medical history is a crucial step in the diagnostic procedure. FXS is a genetic condition, and a family history of intellectual or developmental disabilities, autism, or other related conditions may arouse suspicion.

3. Testing Genetics:

• Genetic testing is used to determine the definitive diagnosis of FXS. Two principal kinds of genetic tests are used to diagnose FXS:

• To examine the FMR1 gene on the X chromosome, a blood or saliva sample is extracted, and DNA analysis is performed. The most important aspects of this analysis include:

• The counting of CGG repetitions in the FMR1 gene. Individuals with FXS typically have an abnormally high number of CGG repeats (over 200 repeats).

• Identifying the FMR1 gene's methylation status. Typically, the gene is methylated in FXS, resulting in its inactivation and the absence of the FMRP protein.

• Molecular Testing: Molecular testing can provide specific details about the CGG repeat expansion, including the exact number of repeats and any mutations within the repeats. This data can be used to determine the likelihood of passing on the mutation to future generations.

4. Carrier Testing: Carrier testing may be recommended in families with a history of FXS or in individuals at risk of possessing the FMR1 premutation (between 45 and 200 CGG repeats). Carriers can be identified by a carrier test.

5. Prenatal Testing: Couples at risk of having a child with FXS have access to prenatal testing for the condition. The FMR1 gene in fetal DNA can be analyzed using techniques such as chorionic villus sampling (CVS) or amniocentesis.

6. Some American jurisdictions include FXS as part of their newborn screening programs. This means that infants born in these states will be screened shortly after delivery for the presence of FXS, allowing for early diagnosis and intervention.

7. Individuals with FXS may endure a comprehensive assessment by a team of healthcare professionals, including developmental specialists, speech therapists, occupational therapists, and psychologists, once a diagnosis has been confirmed. This evaluation helps determine the individual's specific requirements and appropriate interventions.

It is crucial to observe that early diagnosis and treatment are essential for managing FXS. Once diagnosed, individuals with FXS can receive individualized support and therapies to address their developmental and behavioral difficulties, potentially enhancing their quality of life and enabling them to reach their maximum potential. In addition, genetic counseling can inform families about the pattern of inheritance and the risk of FXS in future pregnancies.

Comprehending The Molecular Foundation

Fragile X syndrome (FXS) is caused by a genetic mutation influencing the FMR1 gene, which is located on the X chromosome. To comprehend the molecular basis of FXS, it is essential to investigate the specific genetic alterations and their effects.

1. CGG Repeat Enlargement:

• The FMR1 gene typically contains a cluster of CGG (cytosine-guanine-guanine) repeats in a particular region. This CGG repeat region typically contains fewer than 45 repeats in individuals without FXS.

2. Change in FXS:

• There is an aberrant expansion of the CGG repeat region in the FMR1 gene in FXS patients. This expansion may involve hundreds or even thousands of CGG repeats, which is significantly higher than the norm.

• There is a correlation between the extent of the repeat expansion and the severity of the syndrome. Larger repeat expansions are associated with more severe symptoms.

3. Methylation and Silencing of Genes:

• One of the critical molecular mechanisms in FXS is the methylation of the FMR1 gene.

• The CGG repeat region becomes hypermethylated when its size exceeds a certain threshold (typically 200 repeats). Methylation is the addition of methyl groups to

DNA, which effectively silences the gene.

- Hypermethylation of the FMR1 gene results in its inactivation, indicating the gene is unable to produce the FMRP (Fragile X Mental Retardation Protein) normally produced in individuals without FXS.

4. Protein Deficiency in FMRP:

- FMRP is an indispensable protein that regulates synaptic plasticity and protein synthesis in the brain.

- The absence or deficiency of FMRP owing to gene silencing disrupts normal brain development and function in FXS patients. Several cognitive and behavioral symptoms associated with FXS are believed to result from this disruption.

5. Neurological Consequences:

• The absence of FMRP in the brain impairs the communication and adaptation of neurons to new information. This disruption in synaptic plasticity can result in learning problems, intellectual disability, and cognitive impairments.

6. Behavioral and Cognitive Signs and Symptoms:

• The molecular changes in the FMR1 gene are responsible for the broad array of behavioral and cognitive symptoms observed in individuals with FXS, including social anxiety, repetitive behaviors, sensory hypersensitivity, and speech and language difficulties.

7. Physical Attributes:

• While FXS predominantly affects the brain and behavior, mild physical characteristics such as a long face, large ears, and a prominent jaw or forehead may also be present. However, these characteristics are typically less pronounced than those seen in other genetic syndromes.

Understanding the molecular basis of FXS provides insight into how the genetic mutation manifests clinically.

It also contributes to the development of potential treatments and interventions aimed at addressing the underlying molecular and neurological abnormalities associated with FXS.

Researchers continue to investigate therapeutic strategies, such as medications and genetic therapies, to mitigate the effects of this genetic disorder and enhance the quality of life of FXS patients.

CHAPTER THREE
Management And Treatment

Treatment and management of Fragile X syndrome (FXS) are typically individualized to address the unique requirements and difficulties of each affected individual.

FXS is a complex disorder characterized by a wide range of symptoms; therefore, a multidisciplinary approach involving healthcare professionals from a variety of disciplines is often recommended.

Here are some important aspects of FXS treatment and management:

1. Early diagnosis and intervention are essential for FXS patients. Early intervention services, such as speech therapy, occupational therapy, and developmental interventions, can aid in the treatment of developmental delays and difficulties with communication and motor skills.

2. Educational Presentation:

• Children with FXS frequently need specialized educational assistance. Individualized education programs

(IEPs) and educational accommodations can assist in customizing the learning environment to the student's particular requirements. Programs for special education may be necessary.

3. Psychological and Behavioral Therapies:

• Behavioral interventions, such as applied behavior analysis (ABA), can be effective in addressing difficult behaviors and imparting adaptive skills.

• Psychological counseling and therapy may aid FXS patients and their families in coping with anxiety, mood disorders, and social challenges.

4. Medical treatments:

• Medication may be prescribed for the management of specific symptoms and related conditions. For instance, stimulant medications may be prescribed to treat symptoms of attention-deficit hyperactivity disorder (ADHD), whereas selective serotonin reuptake inhibitors (SSRIs) may be used to treat anxiety and mood disorders.

5.   Sensory   Integration Counseling:

• Some individuals with FXS have heightened sensory perception. Therapy for sensory integration can help them adapt to sensory input and increase their tolerance for a variety of sensations.

6. Support for Speech and Communication:

• Speech and language therapy can help individuals with FXS improve their verbal and nonverbal communication abilities.

7. Social Skills Instruction:

• Individuals with FXS may benefit from social skills training to improve their social interactions and reduce social anxiety.

8. Counseling for Genetic Considerations:

• Genetic counseling can provide families with information and support about the inheritance pattern of FXS and the likelihood of having additional affected children.

9. Services of Assistance and Advocacy:

• Support groups and advocacy organizations can offer families affected by FXS emotional support and resources. They can also help raise awareness of the condition and promote research into it.

10. Investigation and Clinical Tests:

• Participation in clinical trials and research studies can provide access to new treatments and therapies for FXS. Research is ongoing, and new approaches are being investigated.

11. Family Education and Adaptation Techniques:

• Families of individuals with FXS benefit from education about the condition and coping strategies for addressing the difficulties it presents. This can assist in strengthening family dynamics and resiliency.

12. Transition Preparation:

• Transition planning becomes essential as individuals with FXS enter adolescence and maturity. There may be a need for preparation for independent living, vocational training, and ongoing support services.

Noting that FXS is a lifelong condition is essential, as treatment and management strategies may need to be modified over time to accommodate changing requirements and abilities.

Individuals with FXS can live fulfilling lives and realize their full potential with the assistance of a coordinated, individualized approach and strong family support. In addition, ongoing research on FXS may one day lead to the development of novel therapeutic options.

Being Affected By Fragile X Syndrome

Fragile X syndrome (FXS) can present affected individuals and their families with both unique challenges and opportunities. While the severity of the condition differs from person to person, there are a number of important factors to consider when discussing life with FXS:

• Individual Variations FXS is a highly variable condition, and no two FXS patients are identical. Even among siblings with the same genetic mutation, the severity and combination of symptoms can differ widely.

• Early Diagnosis and Intervention: Early diagnosis and intervention are crucial. Access to early intervention services, specialized education, and therapies can significantly enhance the developmental outcomes of an individual. Early intervention can aid individuals with FXS in acquiring vital skills and enhancing their quality of life.

• Creating a supportive and empathetic atmosphere is essential. Family members, caregivers, and educators can play a crucial role in assisting those with FXS to navigate daily life and realize their complete potential. Important are patience, empathy, and a willingness to adapt to the individual's requirements.

• Numerous individuals with FXS benefit from speech therapy, occupational therapy, behavioral interventions, and training in social skills. These therapies can assist with communication difficulties, sensory sensitivity, and behavioral difficulties.

• Some individuals with FXS may require medications to manage symptoms such as anxiety, hyperactivity, and mood disorders.

The administration of medications should be strictly monitored by medical professionals.

• Social and Emotional Support: Individuals with FXS may struggle with social anxiety and interpersonal difficulties. It is crucial to provide opportunities for socialization and support for anxiety management. Mental health professionals and support groups can provide invaluable assistance.

• Vocational and Independent Living Skills are essential components of transition planning for adolescents and young adults with FXS. Individuals can attain greater independence through vocational training, the development of independent living skills, and ongoing support services.

• Living with FXS can have an effect on family dynamics. Parents and children may face unique challenges and growth opportunities. Beneficial are open communication within the family and support from FXS advocacy organizations.

• Advocacy and Awareness: Advocacy is essential for increasing FXS awareness and promoting research into the condition. Numerous families and individuals with FXS become advocates to increase community understanding, access to resources, and support.

• It is essential to observe that FXS research is ongoing and that new therapeutic approaches and treatments are being investigated. While there is no cure for FXS, advancements in science and medicine offer hope for a better quality of life for those affected.

• Celebrating milestones and accomplishments, regardless of their size, is crucial. Recognizing and celebrating a person's advancements and achievements can enhance self-esteem and motivation.

Individuals with FXS can lead meaningful and fulfilling lives if they have adequate support, resources, and a positive outlook. Families and caregivers can play a vital role in assisting people with FXS to flourish and overcome obstacles by emphasizing their unique abilities and strengths.

Perspective And Conclusion

Over the years, the prognosis for individuals with Fragile X syndrome (FXS) has improved due to advances in research, early intervention, and supportive services. Despite the fact that FXS is a lifelong condition that presents obstacles, there is cause for optimism:

• Early Intervention: Early diagnosis and intervention are crucial for enhancing the prognosis of FXS patients. Early access to therapies, educational assistance, and behavioral interventions can significantly improve developmental outcomes and quality of life.

• Individual Progression: Every person with FXS is unique, and their progression and potential vary greatly. With the appropriate support and interventions, numerous people with FXS make significant gains in communication, social skills, and independence.

- Advancements in Research: Ongoing FXS research continues to shed light on the disease's underlying biology and potential therapeutic approaches. While there is no cure for FXS, research may contribute to the development of innovative treatments and therapies that target the condition's underlying causes.

- The FXS community consists of a close-knit network of individuals, families, caregivers, and advocacy organizations. These communities offer invaluable emotional support, resources, and connection opportunities.

• Awareness and Advocacy: Increased awareness of FXS and advocacy efforts have led to enhanced access to services, funding for research, and policies that benefit individuals with the condition.

Despite the fact that Fragile X syndrome presents enduring challenges, individuals with FXS and their families can live fulfilling lives with the appropriate interventions and support. A positive outlook requires a prompt diagnosis, individualized treatments, and a positive, nurturing environment.

As FXS research continues, there is optimism that new remedies and therapies will further improve the quality of life of those affected by this condition. Individuals with FXS are capable of achieving significant milestones and making contributions to their communities.

THE END

www.ingramcontent.com/pod-product-compliance
Lightning Source LLC
Chambersburg PA
CBHW060808260726
48660CB00002B/841